A PRACTICAL INTRODUCTION

TO MAJOR

CHINESE HERBAL FORMULAS

Dr. Hong-yen Hsu
Douglas H. Easer

Oriental Healing Arts Institute

Educational Series on Chinese Medicine
Number One

A PRACTICAL INTRODUCTION TO
MAJOR CHINESE HERBAL FORMULAS

ISBN: 0-941 942-00-7

Table of Contents

Notice

The following is a summary description of some of the natural herbal formulas widely used throughout Asia. The information compiled from traditional medical texts and from the observations of modern authorities on Chinese medicine is presented here for its educational value and should not be used for diagnosis, treatment, or prevention of disease without the advice of a Chinese physician or other medical authority.

Foreword

The study of natural history in the West dates from the time of Hippocrates (460-370 B.C.). Dioscordes, a Greek physician who lived in the first century A.D., wrote *De Materia Medica* in A.D. 78. He described about six hundred plants that were known to have medicinal properties. In contrast, the origins of Chinese medicine may very well date back to prerecorded history with the earliest written medical references found in the *Tso chuan*, the chief historical source of the Spring and Autumn period in China (722-481 B.C.). The first book of pharmacology in China, *Shen Nung's Herbal* (*Shen nung pen ts'ao ching*), was published during the Han dynasty (206 B.C. - A.D. 220) and described 365 drugs: 252 of plant origin; 67 of animal origin; and 46 of mineral origin.

Chinese medicine still relies upon herbal therapy (herbs, roots, and tonics) as essential to diagnosis and prognosis of disease. Based on an empirical system, it uses only natural drugs and effectively treats many chronic and degenerative diseases without the side effects that plague many Western medicines. Chinese herbal medicine is used by more than one billion people throughout Asia today.

The Oriental Healing Arts Institute was established in response to two long-term developments: (1) the demonstrated effectiveness of Chinese herbal medicine; and (2) the inability of Western medicine, despite the use of drugs and surgery, to stem the tide of chronic and degenerative illnesses sweeping the industrialized world. Put another way, it seems unfortunate that therapies that have demonstrated their effectiveness for more than two thousand years and are providing one-fourth of the world community with most of its common remedies should be limited to China.

The Institute is a nonprofit educational organization devoted to introducing and furthering research and understanding of Chinese medicine. Current efforts include the publication of a bi-monthly bulletin and of classical and modern works of Chinese medicine. This is the first time that a systematic effort has been made in the West to translate some of the major works of Chinese medicine from the hundreds of publications released annually.

The Institute's Educational Series on Chinese Herbal Medicine is designed to acquaint the reader with the effectiveness of commonly used Chinese herbs and herbal formulas in treating disease. The first publication of this series is entitled "A Practical Introduction to Major Chinese Herbal Formulas." The projected second publication is "Gynecological Disorders and Their Chinese Herbal Treatment." The purpose of the series is to help the reader become aware of proven herbal remedies that are natural products and readily available in the United States. If this series contributes to a growing awareness of the effectiveness of Chinese herbal therapy, then my goal has been fulfilled.

Hong-yen Hsu, Ph.D.
Los Angeles, California
June, 1980

Preface

Chinese Medicine Today

This manual provides an introduction to Chinese medicine and some of the commonly used Chinese herbal formulas. The main part of the text is divided into twelve disease categories. Each category lists the most effective formulas for treating that specific type of disease. Below each herbal formula the following items are listed: herbal components; actions of the herbs; and uses or application.

Mention is made of herbal formulas which are approved for use in medical clinics by the Japanese government or the National Health Administration of Taiwan or both. When we speak of Chinese medicine we are speaking of a living tradition, not one which has been supplanted by Western medicine. Some of the same formulas are mentioned in numerous sections; it is hoped that this will prove a testimony to their versatility and effectiveness. A brief definition accompanies the most obscure medical terms found in the text and a glossary of the herbal formula components is provided in the appendix. Naturally, because some herbal formulas are mentioned more than once and the same medical terms occur throughout the text, there is some repetition, but it was felt that such a format would improve the readability of the material.

People in the United States are becoming more health conscious while at the same time public confidence in modern medicine is drastically declining, giving rise to a search for alternative therapies. Recent interest in Chinese medicine has grown tremendously and its use is being revived throughout Asia. Research and training in Chinese medicine is carried on in the countries of China, Taiwan, and Japan, offering the patient an alternative to modern Western medicine.

In the People's Republic of China, the government since 1949 has actively encouraged scientific research in Chinese medicine. In 1958 the Chinese Academy of Medical Sciences in Peking established the Institute of Materia Medica to conduct scientific research on herbal drugs in order to develop new methods for the treatment of common diseases. Furthermore, beginning in 1970 the government required all medical schools to teach Chinese as well as Western medicine. Currently there are 280,000 licensed Chinese physicians; those trained in Western medicine exceed 360,000. In addition, 1,600,000 "barefoot doctors" (paramedics), 10,000 of whom are being trained annually, prescribe and adminster common herbal remedies. The basic reference work used by these paramedics is *The Barefoot Doctor's Manual,* which lists more than 500 commonly used herbal medicines. At least one-half of the population uses Chinese medicine supplied by over 40,000 drug stores usually carrying an inventory of 800 to 900 different products.

Taiwan, an area about the size of Rhode Island, has a population of more than 17,000,000. The total number of Chinese drug stores serving this area is 6,918. Besides these pharmacies, 289 herb shops deal exclusively in the sale of raw herbs. Over one thousand, six hundred physicians practice herbal medicine. Anyone aspiring to become a

Chinese physician must graduate from the Chinese Medical College in Taichung and graduates must pass a rigorous set of examinations in order to obtain a Chinese physician's license. For example, of the more than six thousand applicants who took the most recent examination, less than 1 percent passed. A number of research organizations and universities conduct research in Chinese medicine in Taiwan, including the Brion Research Institute of Taiwan, the National Taiwan Medical School, and Taipei Medical College. It is evident that the art of practicing Chinese medicine in Taiwan is tightly controlled to ensure quality care.

Chinese medicine was first introduced in Japan during the Chin dynasty (221-207 B.C.) but it was not until the seventh century that it took hold. Chinese medicine maintained its supremacy until the nineteenth century when it was superseded by European medicine. However, after World War II interest in Chinese herbal medicine revived. Beginning in 1969, several organizations and departments in private and public universities were established to conduct research in this field. In 1976 a law was passed enabling people to obtain certain herbal prescriptions under the National Health Insurance system. The National Health Department of the Japanese government currently has approved 220 different kinds of medicinals for use in clinics. Some twenty to thirty thousand Japanese physicians trained in Western medicine use Chinese herbal formulas in addition to modern methods to treat their patients, and Japanese consumers spend more than $2,000,000,000 annually on Chinese medicinals.

Traditionally, Chinese herbal medicine has been decocted; that is, the ingredients of a particular herbal formula are placed in 500 grams of water which is then brought to a boil and allowed to simmer for one to two hours. One saying goes that the more bitter the taste the better the formula. In 1954 the Sun Ten Pharmaceutical Company of Taiwan began to produce scientifically formulated herbal combinations in powder, granule, pill, and capsule form. This method is preferable to decoction because it ensures maximum potency of the formula, and makes medication more convenient and palatable. The herbal formulas mentioned in this manual may be decocted or purchased in powder, granule, pill, or capsule form.

Introduction

Scientific progress and medical advancements have brought material comforts to man and extended his life span. Yet despite medical progress, modern medical science has been almost powerless to cope with the rising tide of degenerative diseases that plague the industrial world. Technological advancement has been accompanied by many unforeseen consequences that are harmful to human health, such as air pollution, adulteration of foods, and drug toxicities. Factories discharge large amounts of waste matter daily which often include poisonous cyanides and mercurides. Adulteration of foods results from insecticides and additives such as artificial colorants, preservatives, artificial sweeteners, and antioxidents, which are used to preserve a fresh appearance and flavor. Statistical evidence indicates that the average individual consumes more than one hundred different additives daily. Modern medicine is effective in treating acute diseases, but drugs such as penicillin, adrenocorticotropic hormone, tetracycline, and many others have serious side effects harmful to the human body. Chronic and degenerative diseases on the increase are cancer, asthma, high blood pressure, arteriosclerosis, chronic hepatitis, rheumatism, diabetes mellitus, kidney ailments, uremia, and heart disease. Thus far modern medical science has not developed successful therapeutic methods for curing these diseases; however, Chinese medicine when applied to these diseases either cures or significantly reduces the pain.

The basic theories of Chinese medicine are found in the *Yellow Emperor's Classic of Internal Medicine* (*Huang ti nei ching*), the *Treatise on Febrile Diseases* (*Shang han lun*), and *Summaries of Household Remedies* (*Chin kuei yao lueh*). The latter two were written nearly two thousand years ago by Chang Chung-ching. Chang is often spoken of as the Chinese Hippocrates and venerated as the Sage of Medicine. Since that time these theories have evolved into Chinese medicine as it is practiced today. The basic principles of treatment are derived from the theory that diseases occur as a consequence of imbalance between normal vitality and toxic substances which have accumulated in the body.

Chinese and Western Medicine Compared

Modern medical science is highly analytical and by reducing the body to its component parts, it devises appropriate therapy based on experimental studies of bacteriology, physiology, and pharmacology along with clinical research. Practitioners of modern medicine concentrate on identifying the disease by isolating it to a single cause, then healing that specific area of the body. The proper medicine cannot be prescribed if the illness is unknown or undecided. The drugs used in treatment are composed of synthetic and chemical substances and surgery is employed as a principal tool. Moreover, medicines are prescribed without consideration of the patient's constitution and life style, or of environmental factors such as climate.

Chinese medicine in contrast is intertwined with a philosophical and metaphysical view of life based on comprehensive whole body treatment. The Chinese physician does not need to know the name of the illness in modern medical terms. Rather, he pays special attention to the patient's subjective complaints or conformation and prescribes a holistic treatment on a subjective basis. In short, while modern medicine relies on accurate diagnosis by naming the disease and its causes, Chinese medicine stresses the patient's reactions and approaches the treatment of disease from the standpoint that each individual is unique.

A leading authority on Chinese herbal medicine, Dr. Yakazu Domei, lists the following differences between Chinese and Western medicine:

Chinese Medicine	Western Medicine
1. Philosophical	1. Scientific
2. Synthetic	2. Analytical
3. Holistic	3. Topical
4. Internal	4. Surgical
5. Conformational	5. Heteropathic
6. Empirical	6. Theoretical
7. Hygienic	7. Preventive
8. Individual	8. Socialized
9. Preventive	9. Bacteriological
10. Experiential	10. Experimental
11. Humoral	11. Cellular
12. Subjective	12. Objective
13. Natural sources	13. Synthetic analogs

Chinese medicine regards the universe as an organism and man as a microcosm of the universe. Western medicine views the human body as a machine or mechanism made up of component parts and develops its theories from this assumption. These different assumptions have created or led to the differences between Chinese and Western medicine.

From the above description it is evident that Chinese medicine is holistic in approach. For example, if a patient's eyes are red, a Western doctor will use lotion to wash the eyes while the Chinese physician will regard the disorder as "overthriving fire" and try to reduce the fire in the patient by having him take such fire-dissipating agents as coptis or gardenia. Another example is the treatment of itching skin, a condition related in Chinese medicine to the vitality of the liver, making the liver the focal point for treatment. The Western physician would more than likely use a dermatological lotion to cure a skin ailment, focusing on the specific symptom rather than its cause.

Chinese medical theory holds that diseases are brought about by either internal or external causes. External causes arise mainly from geography, weather, and environment and are known as the "six excesses," namely, wind, dryness, cold, fire, moisture, and heat. Internal causes are the

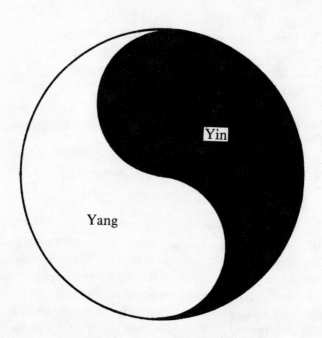

Fig.1 Yin/yang Theory: The Fundamental
Principle of Chinese Medicine

"seven emotions," namely, joy, anger, sorrow, brooding, grief, fear, and shock. The progress of disease varies with an individual's constitution, temperament, site of the symptoms, nutrition, and circulation of the blood, water, and *ch'i* (physiological energy). According to the famous *Treatise on Febrile Diseases,* the various stages of disease are known as the "six paths": greater yang, lesser yang, sunlight yang, lesser yin, greater yin, and absolute yin (See Figure 2). Different herbal formulas are used for the different stages of the disease. Disease conformations are classified into "excessive" or "deficient." Body conditions are described as "thriving" or "deteriorated," "strong" or "weak." There are eight types of conformation: yin, yang, external, internal, cold, fever, weak, and firm. Once the conformation is decided upon, corresponding herbal formulas are administered.

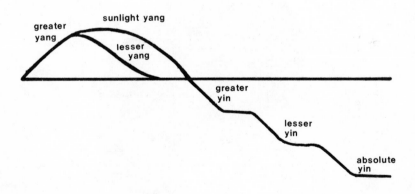

Fig. 2 Six Pathological Stages

The Seven Emotions

Conformations resulting from the seven emotions are mainly diseases of *ch'i* (energy) but they may affect the blood. Diseases related to the seven emotions are internal. Excessive emotional stimulation or inhibition causes imbalances which injure the viscera (internal organs of the body, especially of the thorax and abdomen) thereby inducing disease. *Ch'i* flows through all living things and concentrates along the acupuncture meridians. *Ch'i* diseases affect the nervous symstem and mind and include such diverse conditions as schizophrenia and Parkinson's disease. For example, pleasure calms *ch'i*, grief diminishes *ch'i*, anxiety obstructs *ch'i*, fear supresses *ch'i*, terror disturbs *ch'i*, brooding coagulates *ch'i*, and anger stimulates *ch'i*. Violent anger injures yin and agitates the blood. The seven emotions cause visceral diseases via the heart because the heart governs the viscera. (See Fig. 3)

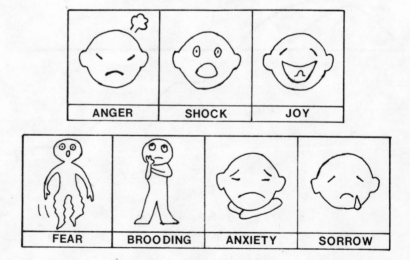

Fig. 3   Seven Emotions

The Five Element Theory

The seven emotions closely interrelate with the five elements, namely, metal, wood, water, fire, and earth. The five elements are in turn mutually interlinked, sometimes reciprocally producing and destroying each other. The five element theory is essential to diagnosis, since bodily functions, organs, acupuncture meridians, emotions, and external factors are related to the various elements. (See Fig. 4) For example, an imbalance in earth may result from an imbalance in wood via the creative cycle, or a deficiency in metal coupled with an excess in earth may necessitate

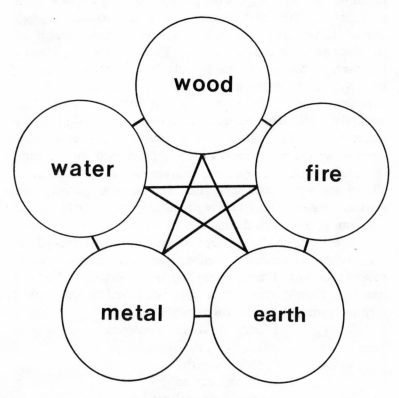

Fig. 4 The Five Element Theory

7

the use of an herbal tea to reduce the energy of earth. The approach to be taken depends upon the patient's diagnostic profile, the symptoms, the pulse diagnosis, and the history of the complaint.

The Four Essences and the Five Flavors

Chinese physicians have experimented with herbal formulas and their effects on the human body for thousands of years. As long as two thousand years ago *Shen Nung's Herbal* (*Shen nung pen ts'ao*) advanced the concept of the four essences and five flavors. The four essences classify the various foods and medicinals into cool, warm, cold, and hot. Diseases with fever as a symptom are treated with medicinals that have cold or cool properties. Alternately, chill diseases with cold limbs as a symptom are treated with medicinals which have hot or warm properties. Herbals with cold properties are gypsum and mirabilitum; those with cooling properties, chrysanthemum and moutan. Medicinals with hot properties are aconite, ginger, and asarum; those with warm properties are *tang-kuei* and cnidium. A neutral medicinal is licorice.

According to the concept of the five flavors, everything that we eat is considered either sour, bitter, salty, sweet, pungent or hot. Bland or no flavor is recognized but not counted. Each flavor has a specific function and action verified through long clinical experience.

Sour:	schizandra seeds, terminalia; astringent action
Bitter:	coptis, rhubarb; fortifying action
Salty:	seaweed, mirabilitum; softening action and expectorant

Sweet: ginseng, rhemannia;
mild strengthening and supplementing actions

Pungent: ginger, perilla;
dispersing action

Bland: hoelen, tetrapanax;
diuretic action

Chinese medicine relates the actions of herbs with the various viscera. This relationship is called the meridian assortment: pungent tasting herbs are associated with the lung; sour tasting herbs, with the liver; bitter tasting herbs, with the heart; and salty tasting herbs, with the kidney. Classification by meridian is equivalent to *in vivo* metabolism in Western medicine.

Although Chinese physicians have studied herbal actions through observation and experimentation for thousands of years, their chemical properties had not been scientifically verified until recently. Pharmacological analysis of Chinese herbal formulas is very difficult because they consist of from four to twelve components. Therefore, until the constituents of the component herbs making up the formula can be broken down pharmacologically, their therapeutic mechanisms cannot be scientifically explained. Only recently have Chinese researchers operating within the framework of the scientific method reported significant findings regarding herbal medicines and their pharmacological actions.

Western medicine classifies medicinals into poisons, potent drugs, and common drugs and studies the pharmacological actions of each drug separately. However, Western medicine emphasizes the healing properties of drugs to the exclusion of their unfavorable side effects, such as allergic reactions or possible inducement of new diseases. Chinese medicine also places herbs and herbal formulas into categories, namely, superior, general, and inferior, based upon the properties and actions of each, but Chinese formulas contain only natural ingredients. Some of the herbs such as *tang-kuei*, lotus seed, and coix

9

are found in the daily diet of the Chinese people. Therefore, most Chinese herbs are compatible with the functions of the human body and capable of being anabolized and absorbed easily.

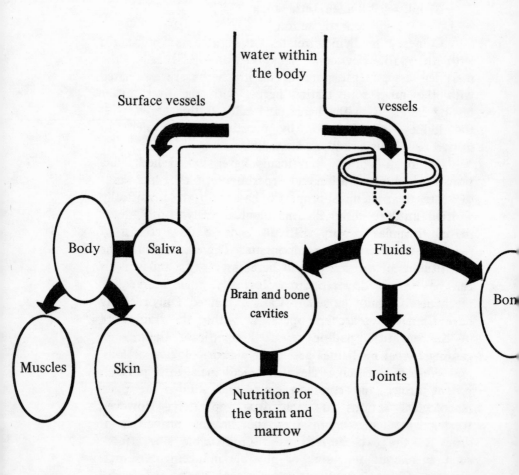

Fig. 5 Distribution of Water Throughout the Body

The Theory of Water, Blood, and *Ch'i*

Many diseases virtually incurable using modern medical methods respond to Chinese herbal medicine. Chinese medicine, as mentioned before, strives to achieve holistic balance in the body by supplementing "weakness" or "emptiness" and by purging "firmness" or "fullness." In conjunction with this approach Chinese medicine classifies diseases as belonging to one humor (a fluid or semifluid part of the body) or another and then devises the appropriate treatment. There are three important humors, namely, water, blood, and *ch'i*. Many diseases are caused by disturbances in water metabolism, an imbalance in circulation, and/or abnormal distribution of water throughout the body. Swelling is the most prominent symptom of water disease but unusual urination or bowel movements or sweating are important signs. Western medicine refers to the action of increasing the flow of urine as diuresis; Chinese herbal medicine refers to it as "water delivery." Many diuretics used in modern medicine have pronounced side effects while Chinese medicine uses gentle-acting water delivering herbs such as hoelen, alisma, atractylodes, and polyporus which are very effective in treating chronic nephritis, uremia and other degenerative diseases. (See Fig. 5) Blood diseases are linked to a malfunctioning circulatory system. Such conditions include blood stagnation, anemia, varicose veins, hardening of the arteries, hemorrhage, and physiological consequences of menstruation and childbirth. In some cases blood stagnation is caused by external injury. (See Fig. 6)

The Japanese call disease *bioki*, literally meaning injured *ch'i*. They believe that disease arises from disturbances in the body and the *ch'i*. *Ch'i* is invisible and omnipresent. Dr. Gonzan Goto, a Japanese authority on Chinese herbal medicine, contends that the obstruction of *ch'i* is the cause of all disease. *Ch'i* can be divided into the mobile and the still. Mobile *ch'i* means up-rushing *ch'i* which

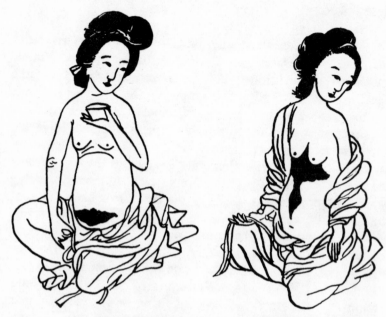

Fig. 6 Types of Abdominal Stagnated Blood

causes dizziness, headache, and "flushing." Cinnamon can be used to suppress up-rushing *ch'i*. For *ch'i* which is obstructed or has accumulated in one place, Chinese herbs such as perilla and magnolia bark are prescribed. Another kind of *ch'i* disease is called the "disease of no disease" and is very difficult to treat with modern Western medicine. Its symptoms are chills, stiff shoulders, habitual constipation, headache, insomnia, giddiness, and hyperemesis gravidarum (excessive vomiting during pregnancy)– all of which are cured fairly easily with Chinese herbal formulas. (See Fig. 7)

Side Effects and Drug Abuse in Western Medicine

Most diseases call for treatment with drugs with the

12

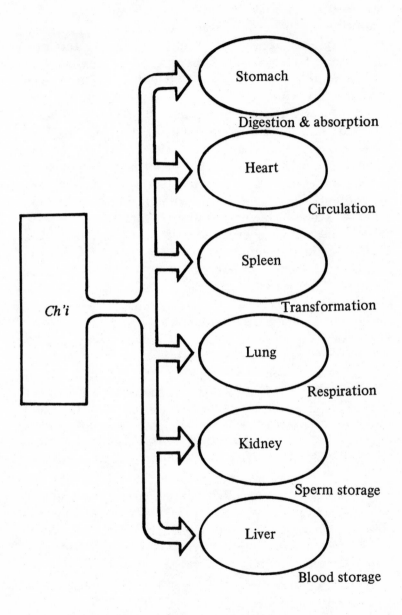

Fig. 7 The Movement of *Ch'i* Through the Body System

exception of those requiring surgery and physical therapy. Despite the fact that drugs are toxic to our bodies, small quantities can be absorbed and disposed of by the body without producing any harmful effects. On the other hand, large amounts of drugs taken continuously over long periods have harmful and cumulative effects resulting in toxic poisoning.

Frequently the administration of drugs results in unintended side effects. According to the World Health Organization, a side effect is defined as: "An ordinary dosage of medicine which leads to an unexpected and harmful reaction." For example, there are several kinds of antibiotics—penicillin and chloramphenicol—which may cause leukemia; adrenocorticotropic hormones may cause aplastic anemia or collagen disease; and other drugs may cause purpura or fulminative hepatitis. All of these diseases are related to the ingestion of drugs per se. Adrenocorticotropic hormone for example is frequently used for the treatment of rheumatism and may cause adrenal atrophy. Antibiotics may inhibit *Streptomyces* or staphylococci but also favor reproduction of *Pseudomonas aeruginosa*, molds, and other types of infectious agents.

As a rule, the fewer number of drugs administered simultaneously, the better. Statistics show that the incidence of side effects from a combination of less than five kinds of drugs is 18.6% whereas six kinds of drugs in combination increase the incidence of side effects to 81.4%. Drugs are first absorbed by the stomach and intestines and then dissociated by the enzymes in the liver or combined with other substances (metabolism) or bound with serum; then they are excreted by the kidneys. Some antibiotics may cause a decrease in intestinal bacteria count, which may in turn cause a disruption of vitamin K production. Then if an anticoagulant is taken, hemorrhage may result.

By way of contrast, when some two hundred varieties of the most commonly used Chinese herbs were extracted with a 50% ethanol solution, the results indicated that the side effects were insignificant. The extracts were forcibly administered to ten male rats in accordance with the Litchfield and Wilcoxon method in order to obtain the LD_{50} values and observe the effects on the central nervous system. Results indicated that the fatality rate of LD_{50} for the majority of herbs was 5g/kg weight. Converted to human dosages this figure would be 250g per 50kg of body weight, which means that 50 percent of a group of people having a body weight of 50kg would die only if they took a dosage of 250g, far above the normal dosage. Thus the side effects or toxicity of Chinese herbs is insignificant at most. It should be added that Chinese physicians have for thousands of years used various processes to reduce toxicity in herbs whenever present.

In sum, Chinese medicine offers all types of cures, from the fundamental to the symptomatic, many of which are not available to modern medical science. Chinese medicine determines the cause of the disease and its effects, and develops a cure that is suited to the uniqueness of each individual. Thus the mental and physical condition of the patient and not the disease is the concern of Chinese medicine. Each herbal formula or tea is intended to treat the general condition of the entire body as well as the specific ailment, working to shore up the body's natural defenses against disease without creating harmful side effects.

TABLE OF SYMPTOMS
AND
THEIR HERBAL REMEDIES

Respiratory Disorders

	Herbal Remedy	Symptoms Treated	Page
1	Pueraria Combination	Common cold--headache, fever, shivering without sweat, shoulder pain	26
2	Minor Bupleurum Combination	Severe cold--lingering cold with mild fever Bronchitis--mild fever, bitter taste in mouth, feeling of fullness in chest, sticky phlegm	27
3	Pueraria and Magnolia Combination	Nasal congestion, chronic rhinitis	28
4	Minor Blue Dragon Combination	Cold with cough--persistent cough with large amounts of phlegm Bronchitis--persistent cough, stridor, watery sputum, congestion, headache, and chest pain	29
5	Pinellia and Magnolia Combination	Harsh cough--moist and harsh cough with itching and pain in throat	30
6	Bupleurum and Cinnamon Combination	Severe cold--lingering cold with mild fever Early stages of tuberculosis, pleurisy with mild fever, and loss of appetite	31

17

Digestive Disorders

Kidney and Gallbladder Disorders

Liver Disorders

	Herbal Remedy	Symptoms Treated	Page
13	Capillaris Combination	Jaundice–fever and constipation	43
11	Capillaris and Hoelen Five Formula	Difficult urination	44
6	Bupleurum and Cinnamon Combination	Hepatitis and jaundice	44

Diseases of Senility

	Herbal Remedy	Symptoms Treated	Page
14	Rehmannia Six Formula	Prostatomegaly (abnormal enlargement of prostate), nephrosclerosis (hardening of renal arteries and arterioles), diabetes, back pain, neuralgia, cataract	46
12	Rehmannia Eight Formula	For same conditions as above but for patient with delicate constitution	47

19

Obesity, Arteriosclerosis, and Hypertension

Gynecological Disorders

Herbal Remedy	Symptoms Treated	Page
19 Bupleurum and Paeonia Formula	Fatigue, tiredness of limbs, chills, vertigo, insomnia, congestion, facial flushing, chilling of back, hot flashes, menopausal disorders	56
20 *Tang-kuei* and Paeonia Formula	Vomiting during pregnancy, heaviness in ear, vertigo, premature labor	57
21 Cinnamon and Hoelen Formula	Headache, vertigo, tinnitus (ringing in one or both ears), chills in lower limbs, congestion, menstrual irregularities in young women	59
22 Persica and Rhubarb Combination	Taken by women of strong constitution with facial redness, headache, vertigo, chilling of lower abdomen, constipation, menstrual disorders	60

Nutrition

Impotence and Problems of Senility

Mental Instability

	Herbal Remedy	Symptoms Treated	Page
28	Ginseng, Longan and B.G. Combination	Emotional instability, nervousness, anxiety, heart palpitations, gastrointestinal weakness	71
5	Pinellia and Magnolia Combination	Neurasthenia, neurosis	72

Joint and Nerve Disorders

	Herbal Remedy	Symptoms Treated	Page
29	Coix Combination	Subclinical arthritis, rheumatism with some pain, swelling and fever; rheumatoid arthritis	74
30	Clematis and Stephania Combination	Chronic sciatic neuralgia, arthroneuralgia, especially below waist	75
12	Rehmannia Eight Formula	Tendency towards fatigue, aching and numbness near waist and in feet	76
1	Pueraria Combination	Primary neuralgia, rheumatism, aching shoulders, facial neuralgia	76

Skin Disorders

Facial Problems

HERBAL FORMULAS
FOR
RESPIRATORY DISORDERS

		Formula(s) No.
1.	Cough	2, 4, 5
2.	Sticky Phlegm	2
3.	Bronchitis	1, 2, 3
4.	Asthma	2
5.	Pneumonia	1, 2, 3, 5
6.	Common Cold	1, 3, 5, 6
7.	Tuberculosis	5
8.	Pleurisy	5, 6
9.	Rhinitis	3
10.	Stridor	4
11.	Chest Congestion	4
12.	Headache	2, 4
13.	Chest Pain	4
14.	Whooping Cough	4
15.	Bronchial Dilation	4
16.	Pulmonary Asthma	4
17.	Influenza	1, 5

1 PUERARIA COMBINATION (*Ko-ken-tang*)

Herbal Compnents

pueraria: 8.0 grams; *ma-huang*: 4.0 grams; cinnamon: 3.0 grams; paeonia: 3.0 grams; jujube: 4.0 grams; licorice: 2.0 grams; ginger: 1.0 gram

Herbs and Actions

Pueraria regulates blood circulation and intestinal function along with bowel evacuation. *Ma-huang* and licorice cure coughs and relieve skin contractions. Paeonia strengthens gastrointestinal function. Licorice detoxifies the liver. Jujube nourishes the body. Ginger, one of the major botanicals in the Chinese materia medica, promotes blood circulation.

This combination was first mentioned in the *Treatise on Febrile Diseases* (*Shang han lun*) and *Summaries of Household Remedies* (*Chin kuei yao lueh*), two Chinese medical classics written in A.D. 205 by Chang Chung-ching, the Chinese Hippocrates.

Uses

Pueraria Combination has been famous in China since ancient times for its curative powers. A physician is considered extremely well-versed in Chinese medicine if he can make full use of this versatile formula. This formula is taken for the common cold, influenza, pneumonia, and bronchitis. The Japanese government has approved Pueraria Combination for use in medical clinics for the common cold.

2 MINOR BUPLEURUM COMBINATION (*Hsiao-chai-hu-tang*)

Herbal Components

bupleurum: 7.0 grams; scute: 3.0 grams; pinellia: 5.0 grams; ginseng: 3.0 grams; jujube: 3.0 grams; licorice: 2.0 grams; ginger: 4.0 grams

Herbs and Actions

Bupleurum and scute are anti-inflammatives and detoxicants, and dispel chest distention. Pinellia and ginger remove fluid accumulated in the stomach, and cure nausea, vomiting, and loss of appetite. A combination of ginseng, jujube, and licorice functions as a stomachic or digestive tonic to relieve the sensations of fullness beneath the heart. Bupleurum nourishes the liver.

Minor Bupleurum Combination was first mentioned in the *Treatise on Febrile Disease* (*Shang han lun*) and the *Summaries of Household Remedies* (*Chin kuei yao lueh*).

Uses

Taken for mild fever, a bitter taste in the mouth, a feeling of fullness in the chest, cough, and sticky phlegm, this natural herbal formula is also useful in treating acute or chronic bronchitis, asthma, pneumonia, headaches, nasal congestion, and the common cold symptom of shoulder stiffness. The Japanese government has approved Minor Bupleurum Combination for use in medical facilities for the common cold or other febrile diseases, bronchitis, tuberculosis, and pleurisy.

3 PUERARIA AND MAGNOLIA COMBINATION (*Ko-ken-chia-hsin-i-chuan-chiung*)

Herbal Components

pueraria: 4.0 grams; *ma-huang*: 4.0 grams; cinnamon: 2.0 grams; paeonia: 2.0 grams; licorice: 2.0 grams; jujube: 3.0 grams; cnidium: 3.0 grams; magnolia flower: 3.0 grams; ginger: 1.0 grams

Herbs and Actions

Pueraria alleviates muscle spasms caused by occluded blood. Licorice coordinates the actions of the other herbs; it functions as a corrective and harmonizing ingredient in a large number of formulas. Ginger regulates vitality. *Ma-huang* and cinnamon increase perspiration. Paeonia and pueraria regulate blood circulation and alleviate muscle spasms. Jujube nourishes the heart and lungs.

This natural herbal combination is mentioned in the *Treatise on Febrile Diseases* (*Shang han lun*) and *Summaries of Household Remedies* (*Chin kuei yao lueh*).

Uses

This combination is taken for the common cold, pneumonia, bronchitis, and rhinitis (inflammation of the nasal mucous membrane).

4 MINOR BLUE DRAGON COMBINATION (*Hsiao-ching-lung-tang*)

Herbal Components

pinellia: 6.0 grams; *ma-huang*: 3.0 grams; paeonia: 3.0 grams; licorice: 3.0 grams; cinnamon: 3.0 grams; asarum: 3.0 grams; schizandra: 3.0 grams

Herbs and Actions

Ma-huang has been used for more than two thousand years to treat headaches, colds, fevers, and skin eruptions. It functions with cinnamon in this formula to remove surface diseases such as severe chills, anhidrosis (deficiency or absence of sweat secretion), and general aching. Cinnamon checks vomiting while *ma-huang* cures cough and stridor (a harsh, vibrating sound produced during respiration). Asarum, ginger, and pinellia relieve ascites (the accumulation of serous fluid in the peritoneal cavity). Pinellia increases the flow of urine. Schizandra, *ma-huang*, asarum, and paeonia are antitussive. Licorice coordinates the actions of the herbs, reduces flushing, and relieves the contraction of tissues.

This natural herbal combination is mentioned in the *Treatise on Febrile Diseases* and *Summaries of Household Remedies*.

Uses

This combination is taken for persistent cough, stridor, watery sputum, congestion, headache, and chest pain. It is also used to treat whooping cough, bronchial dilation, and pulmonary asthma.
Note: This formula is not suitable for those with fragile health and night sweats.

5 PINELLIA AND MAGNOLIA COMBINATION (*Pan-hsia-hou-pu-tang*)

Herbal Compnents

pinellia: 6.0 grams; magnolia bark: 3.0 grams; hoelen: 5.0 grams; ginger: 4.0 grams; perilla: 2.0 grams

Herbs and Actions

Pinellia and hoelen relieve abdominal ascites (accumulation of serous fluid in the peritoneal cavity), cure nausea and vomiting, and increase blood circulation. Magnolia bark reduces abdominal fullness and increases vitality. Perilla has a tranquilizing effect and increases gastrointestinal function. Ginger acts as a diuretic, cures vomiting, increases gastrointestinal function, and coordinates the action of the other herbs.

This natural herbal combination is mentioned in the *Summaries of Household Remedies.*

Uses

This formula is effective in treating the common cold, influenza, pneumonia, tuberculosis, and pleurisy. Pinellia and Magnolia Combination is taken for a moist and harsh cough with a scratchy throat and for pain in the throat.

6 BUPLEURUM AND CINNAMON COMBINATION (*Chai-hu-kuei-chih-tang*)

Herbal Components

bupleurum: 5.0 grams; pinellia: 4.0 grams; licorice: 1.5 grams; cinnamon: 2.5 grams; scute: 2.0 grams; ginseng: 2.0 grams; paeonia: 2.5 grams; jujube: 2.0 grams; ginger: 1.0 gram

Herbs and Actions

This herbal combination consists of a combination of Minor Bupleurum Combination (*Hsiao-chai-hu-tang*) and Cinnamon Combination (*Kuei-chih-tang*). Bupleurum promotes blood circulation in the liver and relieves chest distention and moist heat. Scute dispels heat in the chest and may be given for inflammation of the digestive organs. Ginseng improves the functioning of internal organs and increases appetite. Ginger and pinellia arrest vomiting, decrease expectoration, increase appetite and flow of urine, and dispel edema in the stomach and chest. Cinnamon cures "flushing" and headache. Paeonia stimulates the action of the digestive organs and acts as a nutrient when in combination with jujube, ginger, and licorice.

This combination is also recorded in Chang Chung-ching's two works.

Uses

This natural herbal formula is taken for a lingering cold with mild fever, a common cold, and pleurisy.

31

HERBAL FORMULAS
FOR
DIGESTIVE DISORDERS

		Formula(s) No.
1.	Gastritis	7
2.	Enteritis	7
3.	Indigestion	7, 8, 9
4.	Gastroptosis	7, 8, 9
5.	Gastric Ulcer	7, 8
6.	Duodenal Ulcer	7, 8
7.	Gastroenteritis	8, 9
8.	Gastrectasis	9
9.	Vomiting	8
10.	Malnutrition	8
11.	Gastric Relaxation	9

7 PINELLIA COMBINATION (*Pan-hsia-hsieh-hsin-tang*)

Herbal Components

pinellia: 6.0 grams; scute: 3.0 grams; coptis: 2.0 gram; ginseng: 3.0 grams; jujube: 3.0 grams; ginger: 3.0 grams; licorice: 3.0 grams

Herbs and Actions

Coptis and scute are antipyretics (agents which prevent or reduce fever) that relieve anxiety due to stress. Pinellia and ginger cure ascites (accumulation of serous fluid in the peritoneal cavity) and vomiting. Ginseng and licorice improve gastric function. Licorice and jujube coordinate the actions of the other herbs.

This natural herbal formula is the result of countless centuries of valuable, practical experience. It is mentioned in two Chinese medical classics, the *Treatise on Febrile Diseases* (*Shang han lun*) and *Summaries of Household Remedies* (*Chin kuei yao lueh*).

Uses

This formula is well-known for treating such gastrointestinal diseases as gastritis (inflammation of the stomach), enteritis (inflammation of the intestinal tract), indigestion, gastroptosis (downward displacement of the stomach), gastric ulcer, and duodenal ulcer. The Japanese government has approved the Pinellia Combination for use in Japanese medical facilities for gastroenteritis (inflammation of the stomach and intestines), gastrectasis (dilatation of the stomach), gastroptosis, and gastric ulcer.

8 PINELLIA AND GINSENG SIX COMBINATION (*Pan-hsieh-liu-chun-tzu-tang*)

Herbal Components

ginseng: 4.0 grams; atractylodes: 4.0 grams; hoelen: 4.0 grams; licorice: 1.0 gram; pinellia: 4.0 grams; citrus: 2.0 grams; ginger: 1.0 gram; scute: 3.0 grams; coptis: 3.0 grams; ostrea: 4.0 grams

Herbs and Actions

Pinellia, scute, coptis, ginger, ginseng, and licorice of Pinellia Combination (*Pan-hsia-hsieh-hsin-tang*) are effective for subcardiac distention, vomiting, anorexia (loss of appetite), diarrhea, and ascites (the accumulation of serous fluid in the peritoneal cavity). Ginseng, atractylodes, hoelen, licorice, pinellia, and citrus of Six Major Herb Combination (*Liu-chun-tzu-tang*) are effective for gastrointestinal weakness, ascites, subcardiac distention, anorexia, chills, anemia, and a tendency toward fatigue.

This natural herbal formula is a combination of Pinellia Combination (*Pan-hsia-hsieh-hsin-tang*) and Six Major Herb Combination (*Liu-chun-tzu-tang*) and is used for general gastrointestinal disorders. It was first recorded in *Summaries of Household Remedies.*

Uses

This formula is effective for stomach distention, vomiting, indigestion, and malnutrition. It has also been used to treat acute and chronic gastroenteritis (inflammation of the stomach and intestinal mucosa), gastric ulcer, duodenal ulcer, and gastroptosis (downward displacement of the stomach).

9 HOELEN FIVE HERB FORMULA (*Wu-ling-san*)

Herbal Components

polyporus: 4.5 grams; hoelen: 6.5 grams; atractylodes: 4.5 grams; alisma: 6.0 grams; cinnamon: 3.0 grams

Herbs and Actions

The main ingredient of this herbal formula is polyporus which has a diuretic effect (increases the flow of urine), slakes thirst, and has excellent draining abilities. Alisma, hoelen, and atractylodes relieve fluid accumulation in the stomach, increase the flow of urine, and dispel edema (excessive accumulation of fluid in the tissue spaces). Alisma also cures thirst. Cinnamon dispels surface heat, cures "flushing," and acts in conjuction with the other herbs as a diuretic. The combined effect of the five ingredients is the regulation of the imbalance of the internal fluids through diuresis (increased excretion of urine) and thereby alleviation of all symptoms.

Both of Chang Chung-ching's medical classics refer to this natural herbal formula.

Uses

This formula is effective in treating acute gastroenteritis (inflammation of the stomach and intestinal mucosa), gastrectasis (dilatation of the stomach), gastric relaxation, gastroptosis (downward displacement of the stomach), and indigestion.

HERBAL FORMULAS
FOR
KIDNEY AND GALLBLADDER
DISORDERS

		Formula(s) No.
1.	Nephritis	2, 9, 11, 12
2.	Cholecystitis	2, 10
3.	Gallstones	2, 10
4.	Inflammation of the Gallbladder	10
5.	Uremia	9
6.	Renal Cirrhosis	9, 11
7.	Kidney Contraction or Atrophy	11, 12
8.	Edema	12
9.	Difficulty in Urination	12

2 MINOR BUPLEURUM COMBINATION (*Hsiao-chai-hu-tang*)

See page 27

Uses

This natural herbal formula is effective in treating those patients with chronic nephritis (inflammation of the kidney), cholecystitis (inflammation of the gallbladder), and gallstones.

10 MAJOR BUPLEURUM COMBINATION (*Ta-chai-hu-tang*)

Herbal Components

bupleurum: 6.0 grams; scute: 3.0 grams; pinellia: 3.0 grams; ginger: 4.0 grams; *chih-shih*: 2.0 grams; paeonia: 3.0 grams; rhubarb: 1.0 gram; jujube: 3.0 grams

Herbs and Actions

Bupleurum and scute remove "harmful heat" and distention in the chest. *Chih-shih* and paeonia relieve muscular tenstion and promote digestion. Rhubarb is anti-inflammative. Ginger relieves nausea and vomiting. Pinellia relieves gastric distress and vomiting. Ginger and jujube synthesize and reinforce the action of the other herbs.

This combination was first recorded in the *Treatise*

37

on *Febrile Diseases* and *Summaries of Household Remedies*; it is used for more severe symptoms than those treated by the Minor Bupleurum Combination.

Uses

This formula is effective in treating gallstones and cholecystitis (inflammation of the gallbladder). The Japanese government has approved Major Bupleurum Combination for use in medical clinics for the urological disorders of gallstones and inflammation of the gallbladder.

9 HOELEN FIVE HERB FORMULA (*Wu-ling-san*)

See page 35

Uses

This effective natural herbal formula is used in treating nephritis (inflammation of the kidney) and uremia (a toxic condition resulting from kidney failure). The Japanese government has approved Hoelen Five Formula for treatment of urological disorders such as nephritis (inflammation of the kidney) and renal cirrhosis (interstitial inflammation of the kidneys).

11 CAPILLARIS AND HOELEN FIVE FORMULA (*Yin-chen-wu-ling-san*)

Herbal Components

capillaris: 4.0 grams; cinnamon: 3.0 grams; polyporus: 4.5 grams; hoelen: 4.5 grams; atractylodes: 4.5 grams; alisma: 6.0 grams

Herbs and Actions

Capillaris is an antiphlogistic (an agent which relieves inflammation) and a diuretic (an agent which increases the volume of urine) that is effective for jaundice. Alisma, polyporus, hoelen, and atractylodes remove stagnant water from the stomach and intestines. Alisma and polyporus eliminate excessive thirst. Cinnamon relieves the sensation of surface fever and synthesizes the actions of the other herbs.

This natural herbal formula is the Hoelen Five Herb Formula (*Wu-ling-san*) with capillaris. It was first mentioned in *Treatise on Febrile Diseases.*

Uses

This formula is effective in treating jaundice, nephritis (inflammation of the kidney), and kidney atrophy.

The Japanese government recommends its use for the urological disorders of nephritis and renal cirrhosis (interstitial inflammation of the kidney).

12 REHMANNIA EIGHT FORMULA (*Pa-wei-ti-huang-wan*)

Herbal Components

rehmannia: 8.0 grams; cinnamon: 1.0 gram; aconite: 1.0 gram; hoelen: 3.0 grams; dioscorea: 4.0 grams; alisma: 3.0 grams; moutan: 3.0 grams; cornus: 4.0 grams

Herbs and Actions

The herbs in this natural formula possess astringent (produces contraction of organic tissues), hematinic (increases the hemoglobin content in the blood), and nutritive qualities. Rehmannia is invigorative, tonic, and nutritive. Cornus is invigorative and kidney strengthening, warms the waist and knees, and helps revitalize the male reproductive organs. Dioscorea nourishes the kidneys, relieves hypothermia (subnormal temperature of the body), and helps restore moisture to dry skin. Moutan dispels stagnant blood and alleviates pain. Hoelen relieves ascites (accumulation of serous fluid in the peritoneal cavity). Alisma increases the flow of urine and alleviates continual thirst. Cinnamon assists rehmannia in improving blood circulation and hoelen in preventing "flushing" from the lower abdomen. Aconite increases body temperature, reactivates the functions of degenerated organs, and functions as a diuretic (increases the volume of urine) when combined with hoelen and cinnamon.

Summaries of Household Remedies mentions that this herbal formula may be used for numbness, beriberi, stagnant water in the stomach, diabetes, and gynecological diseases.

Uses

This natural herbal formula is effective in treating chronic nephritis (kidney inflammation), and kidney contraction and atrophy. It is effective for edema and difficulty in urination.

Note: Chinese physicians recommend that patients who have chronic gastrointestinal weakness, frequent diarrhea, marked ascites (accumulation of serous fluid in the peritoneal cavity) and facial flushing with fever not take this formula.

The Japanese government has approved Rehmannia Eight Formula for use in treating cystitis (inflammation of the bladder).

HERBAL FORMULAS
FOR
LIVER DISORDERS

13 CAPILLARIS COMBINATION (*Yin-chen-hao-tang*)

Herbal Components

capillaris: 4.0 grams; gardenia: 3.0 grams; rhubarb: 1.0 gram

Herbs and Actions

Capillaris is an antiphlogistic (an agent which reduces inflammation) and a diuretic (an agent which increases the volume of urine) which is effective for stagnant heat and jaundice. Gardenia is also an antiphlogistic and a diuretic, effective for stagnant heat, jaundice, and distention in the chest near the heart. Rhubarb is a laxative and an antipyretic (reduces or prevents fever).

This natural herbal formula was first mentioned in Chang Chung-ching's two medical classics.

Uses

This formula is effective in treating jaundice and acute hepatitis (inflammation of the liver).

11 CAPILLARIS AND HOELEN FIVE FORMULA (*Yin-chen-wu-ling-san*)

See page 39

Uses

This natural herbal formula is effective in treating jaundice and hepatitis (inflammation of the liver).

6 BUPLEURUM AND CINNAMON COMBINATION (*Chai-hu-kuei-chih-tang*)

See page 31

Uses

Bupleurum and Cinnamon Combination is taken for hepatitis (inflammation of the liver) and jaundice.

HERBAL FORMULAS
FOR
DISEASES OF SENILITY

		Formula(s) No.
1.	Prostatomegaly	14, 12
2.	Nephrosclerosis	14, 12
3.	Diabetes	14, 12
4.	Lower Back Pain	14, 12
5.	Neuralgia	14, 12
6.	Cataract	14, 12
7.	Muscular Weakness	14, 12
8.	Vertigo	14, 12
9.	Nocturnal Emission	14, 12
10.	Frequency of Urination	14, 12
11.	Glaucoma	14, 12
12.	Impotence	14, 12
13.	Nephritis	14, 12
14.	Edema	14, 12
15.	Dysuria	14, 12
16.	Tendency toward Fatigue	12
17.	Chilled Limbs	12
18.	Loss of Vigor	12

14 REHMANNIA SIX FORMULA (*Liu-wei-ti-huang-wan*)

Herbal Components

rehmannia: 6.0 grams; cornus: 3.0 grams; dioscorea: 3.0 grams; alisma: 3.0 grams; moutan: 3.0 grams; hoelen: 3.0 grams.

Herbs and Actions

Rehmannia Six Formula is used mainly for a yin deficiency. (Yin is the force which produces expansion, as of water and air. It is one of the two forces in nature, the other being yang, that are both mutually complementary and antagonistic). Rehmannia is a tonic for the kidneys and increases their blood volume. Cornus warms the liver and strengthens the kidneys while moutan cools the blood and relieves heat. Dioscorea nourishes the spleen and strengthens the kidneys. Hoelen increases the flow of urine, reduces swelling, and removes the moist heat of the spleen. Alisma is both a diuretic (increases the volume of urine) and a tonic for the ears and eyes.

During the Sung dynasty, Chien I (A.D. 1035-1117), known as the first pediatrician of China, isolated cinnamon and aconite from Rehmannia Eight Formula (*Pa-wei-ti-huang-wan*) and formulated Rehmannia Six Formula. The latter is intended for use in treating milder symptoms than that of the former.

Uses

This formula is effective for elderly people with prostatomegaly (enlargement of the prostate), nephrosclerosis (hardening of the renal arteries and arterioles), diabetes, lower back pain, neuralgia, cataract, muscular weakness, vertigo, nocturnal emission, frequency of urination, glaucoma, impotence, nephritis, edema, and dysuria (painful or difficult urination).

12 REHMANNIA EIGHT FORMULA (*Pa-wei-ti-huang-wan*)

See page 40

Uses

This natural herbal formula is taken for a tendency toward fatigue, cold limbs, loss of vigor, numbness, and all of the conditions described above for Rehmannia Six Formula. However, Rehmannia Eight Formula is used for the patient with a delicate constitution.

HERBAL FORMULAS FOR OBESITY, ARTERIOSCLEROSIS, AND HYPERTENSION

	Formula(s) No.
1. Obesity	15, 16, 10
2. Hypertension	15, 16, 17, 18, 10, 12,
3. Arteriosclerosis	15, 16, 17
4. Shoulder Stiffness	15, 10
5. Palpitation	15, 18
6. Habitual Constipation	16, 17
7. Heart Weakness	16
8. Edema	16

15 SILER AND PLATYCODON FORMULA (*Fang-feng-tung-sheng-san*)

Herbal Components

tang-kuei: 1.2 grams; paeonia: 1.2 grams; gardenia: 1.2 grams; cnidium: 1.2 grams; forsythia: 1.2 grams; nepeta (schizonepeta): 1.2 grams; siler: 1.2 grams; mirabilitum: 1.5 grams; *ma-huang*: 1.2 grams; ginger: 1.2 grams; rhubarb: 1.5 grams; atractylodes: 2.0 grams; mentha: 1.2 grams; platycodon: 2.0 grams; scute: 2.0 grams; licorice: 2.0 grams; talc: 3.0 grams; gypsum: 2.0 grams

Herbs and Actions

Siler and Platycodon Formula is complicated, containing some eighteen components. Rhubarb, mirabilitum, and licorice remove food poisons from the stomach and intestines. Siler, *ma-huang*, and ginger increase skin function. Platycodon, gardenia, and forsythia are antiphlogistics (anti-inflammatives) and detoxicants. Schizonepeta and mentha remove internal heat from the head. Atractylodes and talc increase the flow of urine. Scute and gypsum are antiphlogistics and sedatives. *Tang-kuei*, paeonia, and cnidium increase blood circulation.

This formula was first used during the twelfth century. Liu Wan-su, a famous physician of the time, used it quite frequently.

Uses

This natural herbal formula is used to treat obesity, hypertension and arteriosclerosis, constipation which tends to accompany these conditions, shoulder stiffness,

49

"flushing," and heart palpitation. The Japanese government has approved Siler and Platycodon Formula for obesity, habitual constipation, and arteriosclerosis.

Note: Siler and Platycodon Formula is taken by those of obese constitution with constipation. It is especially effective for those whose obestiy is related to overconsumption of meat.

16 STEPHANIA AND ASTRAGALUS COMBINATION
(*Fang-chi-huang-chi-tang*)

Herbal Compnents

stephania: 5.0 grams; astragalus: 5.0 grams; atractylodes: 3.0 grams; licorice: 1.5 grams; jujube: 3.0 grams; ginger: 3.0 grams

Herbs and Actions

Stephania and atractylodes cure edema, stop excessive perspiration, increase the flow of urine, and relieve pain. Astragalus and licorice nourish the skin. Jujube and licorice improve the taste and coordinate the actions of the other herbs. Ginger acts as a stomachic (a substance which stimulates the secretory activity of the stomach).

This herbal combination was first mentioned in *Summaries of Household Remedies.*

Uses

Stephania and Astragalus Combination should be taken by those of obese constitution with flaccid muscles, heart weakness, edema, and a tendency to tire quickly and perspire easily. The majority of such patients are women. This formula is effective in treating obesity, habitual constipation, and arteriosclerosis. The Japanese government has approved the use of this combination for treatment of obesity.

17 COPTIS AND RHUBARB COMBINATION (*San-huang-hsieh-hsin-tang*)

Herbal Components

rhubarb: 2.0 grams; scute: 1.0 gram; coptis: 1.0 gram

Herbs and Actions

All three herbs of this formula are bitter antiphlogistics (reducing inflammations or fever) and laxatives. Rhubarb contains various anthraguinone derivatives (substances responsible for cathartic action) and emodins (irritant cathartics, acting mainly in the large intestine) and a special tannin (tannic acid). Coptis contains berberine, worenine, and coptisine. Combined, they facilitate bile secretion and bowel evacuation, and are sedative and anti-inflammatory. When used clinically, Coptis and Rhubarb Combination produces remarkable effects due to the synergy (combined action of two or more agents) of the Chinese formula, a concept that is difficult to explain in modern pharmacological terms.

This is a natural herbal formula which has been highly recommended by Chinese physicians since it was first recorded in the Chinese medical classic, *Summaries of Household Remedies,* written during the Han dynasty in A.D. 205.

Uses

This formula is taken for prevention of and recuperation from hypertension, arteriosclerosis, habitual constipation, insomnia, neurosis, and mental instability.

The Japanese government has approved Coptis and Rhubarb Combination for stroke, hypertension, insomnia, habitual constipation, spitting of blood, and uterine bleeding.

18 COPTIS AND SCUTE COMBINATION (*Huang-lien-chieh-tu-tang*)

Herbal Components

scute: 3.0 grams; coptis: 1.5 grams; phellodendron: 1.5 grams; gardenia: 2.0 grams

Herbs and Actions

Coptis dispels "internal heat" in the heart, spleen,

and stomach, and relieves palpitations and distention beneath the heart. Scute dispels "internal heat" in the lungs and intestines and reduces inflammation, congestion, hemoptysis (the spitting of blood), and bleeding. Phellodendron is a diuretic and astringent effective for "internal heat" in the kidneys and bladder. Gardenia is a sedative, hemostatic (an agent that arrests hemorrhage), and antiemetic (an agent that prevents or relieves nausea and vomiting).

This natural herbal formula was first mentioned in the *Prescriptions for Emergencies* (*Chou hou pei chi fang*) by the famous Taoist Ko Hung (A.D. 281-341).

Uses

This formula is effective for heart palpitations and hypertension. The Japanese government has approved Coptis and Scute Combination for use in medical clinics for hypertension.

10 MAJOR BUPLEURUM COMBINATION (*Ta-chai-hu-tang*)

See page 37

Uses

Major Bupleurum Combination is taken for hypertension and obesity by those having a strong constitution with symptoms of chest distention, pressure in the chest, constipation, and shoulder stiffness. The Japanese government has approved this formula for use in its medical facilities to treat hypertension and obesity.

12 REHMANNIA EIGHT FORMULA (*Pa-wei-ti-huang-wan*)

See page 40

Uses

This natural herbal formula is effective for hypertension in elderly people with thirst, fatigue, and frequent urination at night. The Japanese government has approved the Rehmannia Eight Formula to treat hypertension.
Note: Chinese physicians recommend that patients who have chronic gastrointestinal weakness, frequent diarrhea, marked ascites (accumulation of serous fluid in the peritoneal cavity), and facial flushing with fever not take this formula.

HERBAL FORMULAS
FOR
GYNECOLOGICAL DISORDERS

19 BUPLEURUM AND PAEONIA FORMULA (*Chia-wei-hsiao-yao-san*)

Herbal Components

tang-kuei: 3.0 grams; paeonia: 3.0 grams; atractylodes: 3.0 grams; hoelen: 3.0 grams; bupleurum: 3.0 grams; moutan: 2.0 grams; gardenia: 2.0 grams; licorice: 2.0 grams; ginger: 1.0 gram; mentha: 1.0 gram

Herbs and Actions

The principal herbs of this formula are *tang-kuei*, paeonia, and bupleurum. *Tang-kuei* is a mild agent for dispelling stagnant (occluded) blood and a hematinic (an agent which tends to increase the hemoglobin content of the blood). For two thousand years paeonia, a mild anticonvulsant and analgesic (pain relieving) agent, and *tang-kuei* have been used to treat blood diseases. Bupleurum, an antipyretic and stomachic (promotes stomach functions) used for chest distention with resistance and pressing pain and alternating chills and fever, is important in treating liver ailments. Gardenia—which is antiphlogistic (counteracts or reduces inflammation or fever), analgesic, and hemastatic—is given for depression, a glowing sensation, jaundice, anxiety, and insomnia. Moutan is a sedative and anticonvulsive given for headache and low back pain; it may also be used for hypertension, inflammation, bleeding, stagnant blood, and gynecopathy (female disorders). Atractylodes and hoelen are stomachics (a substance that stimulates the digestive activity of the stomach) and diuretics (increase the flow of urine). Mentha is a cooling antidepressive and stomachic. Ginger warms the body and promotes blood circulation. Licorice synthesizes the actions of the other herbs.

Both a medical dictionary published in A.D. 1110 and *Standards for Treatment* published in A.D. 1602 indicate that this formula is very effective for gynecological problems such as aches in the arms and legs, dizziness, mental instability, flushing, thirst, insomnia, cardiac and limb fever, and menstrual irregularity.

Uses

This formula is effective for the treatment of menopausal disturbances, menstrual irregularity, and various symptoms due to abortion or salpingotomy (the operation of cutting into a fallopian tube). The symptoms may include emotional instability, irritability, a tendency toward fatigue, headache, constipation, and backache. The Japanese government recommends Bupleurum and Paeonia Formula for menstrual irregularity and menopausal disorders.

20 TANG-KUEI AND PAEONIA FORMULA (*Tang-kuei-shao-yao-san*)

Herbal Components

tang-kuei: 3.0 grams; cnidium: 3.0 grams; paeonia: 4.0 grams; hoelen: 4.0 grams; atractylodes: 4.0 grams; alisma: 4.0 grams

Herbs and Actions

Tang-kuei, a hematinic (an agent which tends to increase the hemoglobin content of the blood) and nutritive agent, synthesizes the actions of the herbs and eases pain. Atractylodes is a diuretic (increases the flow of urine), while cnidium increases vitality and nourishes the blood. Hoelen dispels inner fluid accumulation and is compatible with atractylodes and alisma.

This natural herbal formula has achieved widespread popularity for treating gynecological disorders. It was first mentioned nearly eighteen hundred years ago in *Summaries of Household Remedies.*

Uses

This formula is taken by women of delicate constitution with chills near the waist and in the feet and an underdeveloped uterus and ovaries which cause habitual abortion. *Tang-kuei* and Paeonia Formula is effective for improving blood circulation, and is a body tonic for women with chills. It is also effective in the prevention of miscarriage. The Japanese government has approved this formula for the gynecological disorders of menstrual irregularity and habitual abortion.

21 CINNAMON AND HOELEN COMBINATION (*Kuei-chih-fu-ling-wan*)

Herbal Components

cinnamon: 4.0 grams; hoelen: 4.0 grams; paeonia: 4.0 grams; persica: 4.0 grams; moutan: 4.0 grams

Herbs and Actions

Cinnamon checks "flushing" and coordinates the effects of the other herbs on blood circulation. Hoelen with cinnamon cures abdominal palpitation and functions as a diuretic (increases urine production). Persica removes stagnant (occluded) blood and increases blood circulation. Moutan also removes stagnant blood and increases vitality. Paeonia causes the expulsion of stagnant blood.

The Chinese consider this natural herbal formula very effective in treating gynecological disorders accompanied by blood stagnation (occluded blood). The prescription for Cinnamon and Hoelen Combination is recorded in *Summaries of Household Remedies* published in A.D. 205

Uses

This natural herbal formula is taken for the gynecological disorders of endometritis (inflammation of the uterine lining), ovaritis (inflammation of the ovary), inflammation of the oviduct, uterine myoma (tumor containing muscle tissue), menstrual irregularities, leukorrhea (mucous discharge from the vagina or cervical canal), backache, shoulder stiffness, and headaches. The Japanese government has approved Cinnamon and Hoelen Combination for disturbances caused by menstrual irregularities.

22 PERSICA AND RHUBARB COMBINATION (*Tao-ho-cheng-chi-tang*)

Herbal Components

persica: 5.0 grams; rhubarb: 3.0 grams; cinnamon: 4.0 grams; mirabilitum: 2.0 grams; licorice: 1.5 grams

Herbs and Actions

Persica and cinnamon dispel stagnant blood in the lower abdomen and improve blood circulation. Cinnamon in combination with licorice relieves "flushing." Rhubarb and mirabilitum dispel "internal heat."

Persica and Rhubarb Combination was first mentioned in *Treatise on Febrile Diseases,* the famous clinical manual compiled by Chang Chung-ching some eighteen-hundred years ago. This manual laid down the general principles of symptomatology (the science of symptoms).

Uses

This formula is taken by those of strong constitution with menstrual irregularity and gynecological disorders. The Japanese government has approved this herbal combination for the treatment of disturbances due to menstrual irregularities and menopausal disorders.

HERBAL FORMULAS

FOR

NUTRITION

23 GINSENG NUTRITIVE COMBINATION (*Jen-sheng-yang-jung-tang*)

Herbal Components

ginseng: 3.0 grams; atractylodes: 4.0 grams; astragalus: 2.5 grams; licorice: 1.5 grams; *tang-kuei*: 4.0 grams; paeonia: 4.0 grams; rehmannia: 4.0 grams; hoelen: 4.0 grams; cinnamon: 2.5 grams; citrus: 2.5 grams; polygala: 1.5 grams; schizandra: 1.5 grams

Herbs and Actions

Ginseng, astragalus, atractylodes, hoelen, licorice, and citrus are good for increasing vitality. *Tang-kuei* nourishes the liver. Rehmannia nourishes the kidneys. Schizandra nourishes the lungs. Polygala nourishes the heart, and cinnamon assists in the synergy (the combined effect of two or more organs or agents) of the herbs.

Since time immemorial the Chinese have regarded ginseng, for which this natural herbal formula is named, as a panacea. According to a government formulary written during the Sung dynasty (A.D. 960-1126), this formula may be used for chronic debility, underweight accompanied by pallor, fever with severe chills, general weakness, anorexia (loss of appetite), mental instability, coughing and wheezing, insomnia, night sweats, amnesia, diarrhea, and dark urine.

Uses

This formula is for those of delicate constitution with general weakness and lack of appetite.

24 GINSENG AND TANG-KUEI TEN COMBINATION
(Shih-chuan-ta-pu-tang)

Herbal Components

ginseng: 3.0 grams; astragalus: 3.0 grams; atractylodes: 3.0 grams; paeonia: 3.0 grams; hoelen: 3.0 grmas; rehmannia: 3.0 grams; cnidium: 3.0 grams; cinnamon: 3.0 grams; licorice: 1.0 grams; *tang-kuei*: 3.0 grams

Herbs and Actions

The ginseng, atractylodes, hoelen, and licorice of Major Four Herb Combination *(Szu-chun-tzu-tang)* are potent stomachic, nutritive herbs which improve appetite and increase digestive absorption. *Tang-kuei*, cnidium, paeonia, and rehmannia or *Tang-kuei* Four Combination *(Szu-wu-tang)* are hematinics (agents which help increase the hemoglobin content of the blood) which improve cardiac and liver functions, cure anemia, and improve coarse skin and blood circulation. Cinnamon and astragalus reinforce these actions.

According to a well-known medical formulary published during the Sung dynasty (A.D. 960-1126), this natural herbal formula treats decreased gastrointestinal function, underweight, anxiety, anorexia (loss of appetite), weakness due to prolonged disease, and lack of vitality.

Uses

Ginseng and *Tang-kuei* Ten Combination is a well-known tonic for debility, anemia, loss of appetite, and chronic diseases involving a lack of vitality, The Japanese government and the National Health Administration of Taiwan have approved this combination for use in medical facilities for convalescence following illness (in patients with delicate constitution).

25 GINSENG AND ASTRAGALUS COMBINATION (*Pu-chung-i-chi-tang*)

Herbal Components

astragalus: 4.0 grams; ginseng: 4.0 grams; licorice: 1.5 grams; atractylodes: 4.0 grams; citrus: 2.0 grams; *tang-kuei*: 3.0 grams; cimicifuga: 1.0 gram; bupleurum: 2.0 grams; ginger: 2.0 grams; jujube: 2.0 grams

Herbs and Actions

Ginseng and astragalus nourish the lungs and act as antihydrotics (agents which inhibit sweating). Ginseng and licorice nourish the spleen and the stomach and increase vitality. *Tang-kuei* nourishes the blood and, in combination with astragalus, nourishes the skin. Atractylodes and citrus improve the functioning of the spleen and stomach. Bupleurum and cimicifuga are antipyretics (agents which reduce or prevent fever). Ginger and jujube coordinate the actions of the other herbs.

This natural herbal combination, first prescribed by Li Tung-yuan, one of the great physicians of the thirteenth century, is generally used for treating a weak pulse, general fatigue, mild fever, headache, night sweats, hypotension, hemorrhoids, and loss of appetite.

Uses

This combination, widely adopted by Chinese physicians, is known as the "king of prescriptions" and is commonly used to increase vigor and body strength. It is taken by those having a tendency toward anemia, fatigue, and loss of appetite, as well as being effective in preventing weight loss during the summer. The Japanese government and the National Health Administration of Taiwan have approved Ginseng and Astragalus Combination for use by those of a delicate constitution with delicate digestive systems.

14 REHMANNIA SIX FORMULA (*Liu-wei-ti-huang-wan*)

See page 46

Uses

Rehmannia Six Formula is for milder symptoms than those treated by Rehmannia Eight Formula. It is taken for obesity in old people, weak knees, frequent urination, dysuria (painful or difficult urination), and itching. Rehmannia Eight Formula is also used to treat these conditions.

HERBAL FORMULAS

FOR

IMPOTENCE AND PROBLEMS

OF SENILITY

26 LYCIUM FORMULA (*Huan-shao-tan*)

Herbal Components

anemone: 1.2 grams; dioscorea: 1.2 grams; achyranthes: 1.2 grams; cornus: 1.2 grams; polygala: 1.2 grams; morinda: 1.2 grams; schizandra: 1.2 grams; cistanche: 1.2 grams; broussonetia: 1.2 grams; hoelen: 1.2 grams; lycium fruit: 1.2 grams; rehmannia: 1.2 grams; fennel: 1.2 grams; eucommia: 1.2 grams; jujube: 4.0 grams

Herbs and Actions

Lycium Formula is a nutritive. Cistanche, morinda, and fennel are good for the kidneys and spleen. Rehmannia and lycium fruit nourish the kidneys and increase vigor. Eucommia and achyranthes help the waist and knees and strengthen the kidneys. Hoelen and dioscorea remove moist heat and strengthen the spleen. Dioscorea and schizandra nourish the lungs and end nocturnal emission. Polygala and anemone increase vitality and improve kidney function. Jujube is a tonic and hematinic (an agent that tends to increase the hemoglobin content of the blood) that nourishes the lungs and strengthens the spleen. Broussonetia is a nutritive.

For many years the Chinese have used this natural herbal formula for improving the functions of the heart, kidneys, spleen, and stomach. It is especially effective in increasing vigor.

Uses

This formula is taken for weakness and decreased sexual desire. The National Health Administration of Taiwan has approved Lycium Formula for use in medical facilities to treat both conditions.

27   BUPLEURUM AND DRAGON BONE COMBINATION
(*Chai-hu-chia-lung-ku-mu-li-tang*)

Herbal Components

bupleurum: 5.0 grams; hoelen: 3.0 grams; pinellia: 4.0 grams; rhubarb: 1.0 gram; cinnamon: 3.0 grams; scute: 2.5 grams; jujube: 2.5 grams; ginseng: 2.5 grams; ginger: 2.5 grams; dragon bone: 2.5 grams; ostrea: 2.5 grams

Herbs and Actions

The principal herbs of this formula are bupleurum, dragon bone , and hoelen. Bupleurum purges inner heat in the chest. Dragon bone soothes and sedates feelings of inner agitation. Hoelen is a diuretic (an agent that increases the flow of urine) and can calm the nerves. Bupleurum and scute relieve heat and stagnation in the chest. Dragon bone and ostrea alleviate chest and abdominal palpitations and relieve cardiac hyperfunction, insomnia, and anxiety. Cinnamon cures "flushing." A combination of hoelen, pinellia, and ginger dispels fluid accumulation in the stomach. Rhubarb purges the intestines, draws out infection, and sedates. Jujube and ginger assist and reinforce the actions of the other herbs.

In his *Treatise on Febrile Diseases* written in A.D. 205, Chang Chung-ching (known as the Chinese Hippocrates) commented that the sedative Bupleurum and Dragon Bone Combination is used to harmonize the "surface" and the "interior" and sedate the mind. This formula is also very effective for a tendency toward fatigue.

Uses

This natural herbal combination is taken by those with a normal constitution who are nervous and have tendencies toward fatigue, excitability, congestion, palpitation, and frequent urination.

14 REHMANNIA SIX FORMULA (*Liu-wei-ti-huang-wan*)

See page 46

Uses

Rehmannia Six Formula is taken for impotence. Rehmannia Eight Formula is also for impotence, but Rehmannia Six Formula is for milder cases than those for which Rehmannia Eight Formula is suitable. The Japanese government and the National Health Administration of Taiwan have approved Rehmannia Six Formula for treating impotence. Rehmannia Eight Formula is approved by the Japanese government for the same purpose.

HERBAL FORMULAS
FOR
MENTAL INSTABILITY

	Formula(s) No.
1. Mental Instability	28
2. Mental Exhaustion	28
3. Nervousness	28
4. Anxiety	28, 5
5. Neurosis	5
6. Neurasthenia	5
7. Insomnia	5

28 GINSENG, LONGAN, AND BUPLEURUM COMBINATION (*Chia-wei-kuei-pi-tang*)

Herbal Components

ginseng: 3.0 grams; atractylodes: 3.0 grams; hoelen: 3.0 grams; jujube: 1.0 gram; longan: 3.0 grams; astragalus: 2.0 grams; *tang-kuei*: 2.0 grams; polygala: 1.0 gram; licorice: 1.0 gram; ginger: 1.0 gram; inula: 1.0 gram; zizyphus: 3.0 grams

Herbs and Actions

Ginseng, astragalus, atractylodes, hoelen, zizyphus, and licorice nourish the spleen and the stomach. Longan, polygala, and jujube nourish the heart and nerves and act as sedatives. *Tang-kuei* treats anemia and, in combination with ginseng, functions as a blood tonic.

A natural herbal formula which was Ginseng and Longan Combination (*Kuei-pi-tang*) with bupleurum and gardenia, was first mentioned in *Formulas for Acute Diseases* (*Chi sheng fang*) by Yen Yung-ho of the Sung dynasty.

Uses

This combination is effective for those of delicate constitution with neurotic symptoms brought on by mental exhaustion, emotional instability, nervousness, and anxiety. The Japanese government has approved this herbal formula for treatment of these conditions.

5 PINELLIA AND MAGNOLIA COMBINATION (*Pan-hsia-hou-pu-tang*)

See page 30

Uses

Pinellia and Magnolia Combination is taken for neurosis, nervousness, emotional instability, neurasthenia, insomnia, and fearfulness (anxiety). The Japanese government has approved this combination for treatment of neurasthenia and neurosis.

HERBAL FORMULAS
FOR
JOINT AND NERVE DISORDERS,
NEURALGIA, ARTHRITIS,
AND RHEUMATISM

	Formula(s) No.
1. Arthritis	29
2. Muscle Aches	29
3. Chronic Sciatic Neuralgia	30
4. Arthroneuralgia	30
5. Rheumatism	29, 1
6. Shoulder Ache	1
7. Facial Neuralgia	1
8. Sciatica	30
9. Aching and Numbness Near the Waist	12

29 COIX COMBINATION (*I-yi-jen-tang*)

Herbal Components

ma-huang: 4.0 grams; *tang-kuei*: 4.0 grams; atractylodes: 4.0 grams; coix: 8.0 grams; cinnamon: 3.0 grams; paeonia: 3.0 grams; licorice: 2.0 grams

Herbs and Actions

Tang-kuei and paeonia promote good blood circulation, synthesize the actions of all the herbs, and relieve pain. Coix alleviates the symptoms of rheumatism, increases the secretion and flow of urine, and dispels accumulated fluid.

The effects of Coix Combination on arthritis and rheumatism have been mentioned in many Chinese medical classics. This natural herbal formula also corrects disturbances in blood circulation, dispels fluid accumulated in the joints and tissues, and relieves muscular tension.

Uses

The formula is effective for arthritis, muscle aches, and especially chronic rheumatic pain. The Japanese government has approved Coix Combination for arthritis, rheumatism, muscular rheumatism, and mucoid arthritis.

30 CLEMATIS AND STEPHANIA COMBINATION (*Shu-ching-huo-hsueh-tang*)

Herbal Components

tang-kuei: 2.0 grams; rehmannia: 2.0 grams; atractylodes: 2.0 grams; cnidium: 2.0 grams; persica: 2.0 grams; hoelen: 2.0 grams; paeonia: 2.5 grams; achyranthes: 1.5 grams; clematis: 1.5 grams; siler: 1.5 grams; gentiana: 1.5 grams; ginger: 1.5 grams; citrus: 1.5 grams; angelica: 1.0 gram; licorice: 1.0 gram; stephania: 1.5 grams; *chiang-huo*: 1.5 grams

Herbs and Actions

Tang-kuei, paeonia, cnidium, and rehmannia make up *Tang-kuei* Four Combination; the addition of persica gives the formula the ability to dispel stagnant blood in the lower abdomen. Hoelen, atractylodes, citrus, *chiang-huo*, angelica, clematis, stephania, and gentiana ease rheumatism in the waist and legs.

Clematis and Stephania Combination was first mentioned in a medical classic published during the Ming dynasty (A.D. 1368-1644). It is well known for increasing blood circulation and for treating rheumatism and severe pain in the muscles, joints, and nerves.

Uses

This formula is taken for chronic sciatic neuralgia (pain along the course of the sciatic nerve), and arthroneuralgia (pain in a joint), especially below the waist. The Japanese government has approved Clematis and Stephania Combination for treatment of neuralgia, sciatica (severe pain along the sciatic nerve), and muscular rheumatism.

12 REHMANNIA EIGHT FORMULA (*Pa-wei-ti-huang-wan*)

See page 40

Uses

Rehmannia Eight Formula is taken for thirst, a tendency toward fatigue, and aching and numbness near the waist and in the feet.

Note: Chinese physicians recommend that patients who have chronic gastrointestinal weakness, frequent diarrhea, marked ascites (accumulation of serous fluid in the peritoneal cavity), and facial flushing with fever not take this formula.

1 PUERARIA COMBINATION (*Ko-ken-tang*)

See page 26

Uses

This formula is taken for neuralgia (severe pain along the course of a nerve), rheumatism, aching shoulders, and facial neuralgia. The Japanese government recognizes this formula as a treatment for neuralgia.

HERBAL FORMULAS
FOR
SKIN DISORDERS

		Formula(s) No.
1.	Eczema	31, 33
2.	Acne	31
3.	Urticaria	31, 32, 1
4.	Carbuncles	31
5.	General Abscesses	31
6.	Furuncles	31, 1
7.	Dermatitis	31
8.	Pruritus	32, 33
9.	Prickly Heat	32
10.	Scabies	32
11.	Itching	33, 1
12.	Coarse Skin	33
13.	Boils	1

31 BUPLEURUM AND SCHIZONEPETA FORMULA
(*Shih-wei-pai-tu-san*)

Herbal Components

bupleurum: 3.0 grams; ginger: 1.0 gram; siler: 2.0 grams; *tu-huo*: 2.0 grams; hoelen: 3.0 grams; platycodon: 3.0 grams; cnidium: 3.0 grams; schizonepeta: 1.0 gram; cherry bark: 3.0 grams; licorice: 1.0 gram

Herbs and Actions

This herbal formula is a detoxicant and reinforces liver function. Bupleurum and ginger promote diaphoresis (perceptible perspiration). *Tu-huo*, siler, and hoelen ease arthritis and rheumatism. Platycodon and cnidium increase the flow of urine and stop suppuration (formation of pus). Schizonepeta and cherry bark are detoxicants. Licorice synthesizes the actions of the other herbs.

The original prescription of Bupleurum and Schizonepeta Formula was modified by a Japanese surgeon. Later a Japanese herbalist added forsythia, after which it became well known as a remedy for skin disorders.

Uses

Recently Dr. D. Yakaju, an authority on Chinese medicine, stated that this herbal formula is especially effective for eczema (a noncontagious, itching skin disease), pimples, and urticaria (hives). It is also used to treat toxic and allergic physical conditions. Continuous application of this remedy in conjunction with 2.0 grams of coix beautifies the skin. Japanese physicians have used this herbal combination to treat carbuncles

78

and general abscesses. Bupleurum and Schizonepeta Formula is also good for furuncles (boils), dermatitis, and acne.

32 TANG-KUEI AND ARCTIUM FORMULA (*Hsiao-feng-san*)

Herbal Components

tang-kuei: 3.0 grams; rehmannia: 3.0 grams; gypsum: 3.0 grams; anemarrhena: 1.5 grams; sesame: 1.5 grams; atractylodes: 2.0 grams; arctium: 2.0 grams; siler: 2.0 grams; akebia: 2.0 grams; licorice: 1.0 gram; cicada: 1.0 gram; sophora: 1.0 gram; schizonepeta: 1.0 gram

Herbs and Actions

Tang-kuei, rehmannia, and sesame nourish the blood. Sophora eliminates "internal heat" in the blood and relieves itching due to scabies. Anemarrhena and gypsum also dispel "internal heat" in the blood and relieve thirst. Arctium and cicada cure "internal heat" and sloughing ulcers. Schizonepeta and siler eliminate "internal heat" and cure scabies. Akebia and atractylodes dispel stagnant blood. Licorice synthesizes the actions of the other herbs.

The Chinese medical work *Orthodox Surgery* (*Wai ko cheng chung*) published in A.D. 1617 indicates that this natural herbal formula was used to treat skin diseases with so-called "internal heat," copious discharge, and pruritus (severe itching).

Uses

This formula is taken for chronic and recalcitrant eczema, chronic urticaria (hives or nettle rash), pruritus (an itching sensation which is a symptom rather than a disease),prickly heat, scabies, and skin diseases aggravated by hot weather. The Japanese government has approved *Tang-kuei* and Arctium Formula for treatment of chronic eczema and urticaria.

33 TANG-KUEI AND GARDENIA COMBINATION (*Wen-ching-yin*)

Herbal Components

tang-kuei: 4.0 grams; rehmannia: 4.0 grams; paeonia: 4.0 grams; cnidium: 4.0 grams; coptis: 1.5 grams; scute: 3.0 grams; phellodendron: 1.5 grams; gardenia: 2.0 grams

Herbs and Actions

Tang-kuei, rehmannia, paeonia, and cnidium of *Tang-kuei* Four Combination nourish the blood and improve liver function. Coptis, scute, phellodendron, and gardenia of Coptis and Scute Combination are refrigerants and detoxifiers that dispel "internal heat" in the blood and in the whole body, and relieve neurotic symptoms and emotional instability.

This natural herbal formula is a combination of *Tang-kuei* Four Combination and Coptis and Scute Combination. It was first mentioned in a medical text written during the Ming period (A.D. 1368-1644).

Uses

This formula is taken for dry eczema, fever, and itching. *Tang-kuei* and Gardenia Combination is effective for skin diseases and for eczema which is associated with an anemic constitution. It is also effective for treating dark brown, coarse skin, and severe pruritus (an itching condition). The Japanese government and the National Health Administration of Taiwan have approved *Tang-kuei* and Gardenia Combination for treating eczema and the thickening and hardening of the skin of the palm of the hand.

1 PUERARIA COMBINATION (*Ko-ken-tang*)

See page 25

Uses

This formula is taken for the early stages of urticaria (hives or nettle rash), inflammation, and itching, as well as furuncles and boils. The Japanese government has approved Pueraria Combination for treating eczema, furuncles, and boils.

HERBAL FORMULAS
FOR
FACIAL PROBLEMS

		Formula(s) No.
1.	Boils	34
2.	Vesicles	34
3.	Eczema	34, 21, 19
4.	Liver Spots	21
5.	Acne	34
6.	Black Spots	21
7.	Urticaria	21
8.	Dermatitis	21
9.	Freckles	21
10.	Facial Pallor	20

34 SILER AND COIX COMBINATION (*Ching-shang-fang-feng-tang-chia-i-yi-jen*)

Herbal Components

schizonepeta: 1.5 grams; coptis: 1.5 grams; mentha: 1.5 grams; *chih-shih*: 1.5 grams; licorice: 1.5 grams; gardenia: 3.0 grams; cnidium: 3.0 grams; scute: 3.0 grams; forsythia: 3.0 grams; angelica: 3.0 grams; platycodon: 3.0 grams; siler: 3.0 grams; coix: 5.0 grams

Herbs and Actions

This formula is made by adding coix to Siler Combination. The purpose of coix is to increase the therapeutic effect of siler, especially when treating facial vesicles (small sacs containing fluid). Coix, scute, and gardenia purge inner heat. Siler, platycodon, and mentha promote diaphoresis (perspiration) and detoxification. Forsythia and *chih-shih* relieve swelling and eliminate pus. Angelica, cnidium, and licorice coordinate and improve the effects of the other herbs. Furthermore, coix has antiphlogistic (reduces inflammation or fever), pus-purging, and analgesic effects.

Shen Chin-ao's *Hygienic Principles* written in A.D. 1773 during the Ch'ing period records: "The Siler and Coix Combination purges anxiety and inner heat of the upper body and cures facial boils and heat diseases."

Uses

This formula is taken for head and facial boils, vesicles, eczema, facial flushing, adolescent acne, and a red nose. The addition of 1.0 gram of coix (*Coicis semen*) each time may produce better results.

20 TANG-KUEI AND PAEONIA FORMULA (*Tang-kuei-shao-yao-san*)

See page 57

Uses

Tang-kuei and Paeonia Formula is taken by women with freckles near the eyes and nose, a delicate constitution, pallor, and a tendency toward fatigue. *Coicis semen* is often added to produce better results. The Japanese government recommends this formula for treatment of black spots.

21 CINNAMON AND HOELEN FORMULA (*Kuei-chih-fu-ling-wan*)

See page 59

Uses

This formula is taken by women with an average constitution for eczema, urticaria (hives or nettle rash), dermatitis, black spots on the skin, pimples, and freckles. The Japanese government has approved Cinnamon and Hoelen Formula for treating eczema and freckles.

19 BUPLEURUM AND PAEONIA FORMULA (*Chia-wei-hsiao-yao-san*)

See page 56

Uses

This formula is taken for eczema, hyperkeratosis (overgrowth of the horny layer of the epidermis), and leukoderma (loss of skin melanin).

35 COICIS SEMEN or COIX (*I-yi*)

See page 83
A derivative of Siler and Coix Combination.

Herbal Components

coix: 30 grams; licorice: 2.0 grams

Uses

This formula is taken for skin abnormalities, frost-bite, and prickly heat.

For further information concerning Chinese herbal medicine, write to the following:

Junkon Medical Industries Co., Ltd.
2-4-8, Uehara, Shibuya-ku
Tokyo 151, Japan

Brion Corporation
12020 B. Centralia Road
Hawaiian Gardens, California 90716
(213) 924·8875-76

Oriental Healing Arts Institute
8820 S. Sepulveda Blvd., Suite 218
Los Angeles, California 90045
(213) 645·9672-94

Sun Ten Pharmaceutical Works Co., Ltd.
114, Chung-Ching South Road, Section 3
Taipei, Taiwan 107

SUGGESTED READINGS

Hsu, Hong-yen and Peacher, William G. *Chinese Herb Medicine and Therapy*. Oriental Healing Arts Institute, Los Angeles: 1976.

Hsu, Hong-yen and Peacher, William G. *Chen's History of Chinese Medical Science.* Oriental Healing Arts Institute, Los Angeles: 1977.

Hsu, Hong-yen. *Chinese Herbs and Formulas.* Oriental Healing Arts Institute, Los Angeles: 1977.

Hsu, Hong-yen. *How to Treat Yourself with Chinese Herbs.* Oriental Healing Arts Institute, Los Angeles: 1980.

Bulletin of the Oriental Healing Arts Institute. Los Angeles, California. Editor: Dr. Hong-yen Hsu.

APPENDIX

A Glossary of Herbs and Their Properties

COMMON NAME	SCIENTIFIC NAME (Family Name)	PART USED	MEDICAL PROPERTIES
Achyranthes	*Achyranthes bidentata* Blume (Amarantha-ceae)	Root	Diuretic, emmenagogue, mucilaginous, demulcent
Aconite	*Aconitum carmichaeli* Debx. (Ranunculaceae)	Root	Stimulant, cardiotonic, analgesic
Akebia	*Akebia quinata* Decne. (Ranunculaceae)	Stem	Diuretic, antiphlogistic
Alisma	*Alisma plantago* L. (Alismataceae)	Stem	Diuretic
Anemarrhena	*Anemarrhena as-phodeloides* Bunge. (Liliaceae)	Rhizome	Antipyretic, expectorant
Anemone	*Anemone cernua* Thunb., *A. pulsatilla* (Ranunculaceae)	Root	Antidiarrheic

Continued

COMMON NAME	SCIENTIFIC NAME (Family Name)	PART USED	MEDICAL PROPERTIES
Angelica	*Angelica dahurica* var. *pai-chi*; *Angelica dahurica* Benth. et Hook. (Umbelliferae)	Root	Aromatic, stimulant, analgesic
Arctium	*Arctium lappa* L. (Compositae)	Fruit	Diuretic, antipyretic, expectorant, antiphlogistic; throat infections
Asarum	*Asarum sieboldi* Miq. (Aristolochiaceae)	Herb	Analgesic, sedative, expectorant; headache, cough, pharyngitis, chronic gastritis, arthritis
Astragalus	*Astragalus hoantchy* Franchet; *A. membranaceus* Bge. (Leguminosae)	Root	Tonic, diuretic, antipyretic
Atractylodes	*Atracylodes ovata* DC. *A. lancea* DC.	Rhizome	Aromatic, tonic; chronic gastroenteritis
Aurantium	*Citrus aurantium* L. (Rutaceae)	Fruit rind	Stomachic, digestant, diaphoretic, expectorant, antitussive, antiemetic
Broussonetia	*Broussonetia papyrifera* Vent. (Moraceae)	Fruit	Stimulant, diuretic, ophthalmic
Bupleurm	*Bupleurum chinense* DC.; *B. falcatum* L. (Umbelliferae)	Root	Antipyretic; nonfunctional amenorrhea
Cherry bark	*Prunus yedoensis* Matsumura (Rosaceae)	Bark	Astringent, antitussive
Chianghuo	*Notopterygium sp.* (Umbelliferae)	Rhizome	Diaphoretic

Appendix

Continued

COMMON NAME	SCIENTIFIC NAME (Family Name)	PART USED	MEDICAL PROPERTIES
Chih-Shih	*Poncirus trifoliata* Rafin. (Rutaceae)	Unripe fruit	Stomachic for dysentery, tenesmus, antidiarrheic
Cicada	*Cryptotympana atrata* Fabr. (Cicadidae)	Exudate	Antipyretic
Cimicifuga	*Cimicifuga dahurica* Maxim. ;*C. foetida* L. (Ranunculaceae)	Root	Antipyretic, sedative, analgesic
Cinnamon	*Cinnamomum cassia* Blume (Lauraceae)	Ramulus	Aromatic, stomachic
Cistanche	*Cistanche salsa* Benth. et Hooker (Orobanchaceae)	Herb	Aphrodisiac, tonic, spermatorrhea; impotence
Citrus	*Citrus nobilis* Lunr. (Rutaceae)	Fruit rind	Stomachic, digestant, expectorant, antitussive, anthelmintic
Clematis	*Clematis chinensis* Osbeck (Ranunculaceae)	Root	Analgesic, rheumatism, antipyretic, diuretic
Cnidium	*Cnidium officinale* Makino; *Ligusticum wallichii* Franch. (Umbelliferae)	Rhizome	Sedative, analgesic, emmenagogue
Coix	*Coix lachryma-jobi* L. (Gramineae)	Seed	Refrigerant, diuretic, antirheumatic; bronchitis, pulmonary abscess, pleurisy, hydrothorax
Coptis	*Coptis chinensis* Franch.; *C. teeta* Wall. (Ranunculaceae)	Root	Bitter stomachic, digestive, antidysenteric
Cornus	*Cornus officinalis* Sieb. et Zucc. (Cornaceae)	Fruit	Astringent tonic in impotence, spermatorrhea, lumbago, vertigo, night sweats

Continued

COMMON NAME	SCIENTIFIC NAME (Family Name)	PART USED	MEDICAL PROPERTIES
Dioscorea	*Dioscorea batatas* Decne. (Dioscoreaceae)	Root	Nutrient tonic, digestant in chronic enteritis and diarrhea; nocturnal enuresis, spermatorrhea, neurasthenia
Eucommia	*Eucommia ulmoides* Oliv. (Eucommiaceae)	Bark	Tonic, sedative and analgesic; hypotension
Fennel	*Foeniculum vulgare* Mill. (Umbelliferae)	Fruit	Carminative, stomachic
Forsythia	*Forsythia suspensa* Vahl (Oleaceae)	Fruit	Antipyretic, antiphlogistic in infectious fevers, suppurative; inflammation, phlegmon, variola, erysipelas, measles
Gardenia	*Gardenia florida* L. *G. jasminoides* Ellis (Rubiaceae)	Fruit	Antipyretic, hemostatic, antiphlogistic in jaundice
Gentiana	*Gentiana scabra* Bunge (Gentianaceae)	Root	Stomachic
Ginger	*Zingiber officinale* Rosc. (zingiberaceae)	Rhizome	Stomachic, stimulant, antiemetic
Ginseng	*Panax ginseng* C.A. Meyer (Araliaceae)	Root	Tonic, stimulant, aphrodisiac, indicated in neurasthenia, dyspepsia, palpitation, impotence, asthma
Gypsum	Gypsum, Native Calcium Sulfate, Alabaster, Selenite, Satinite, Tera Alba	Mineral	Sedative, antipyretic, antiphlogistic
Hoelen	*Poria cocos* Wolf. (Polyporaceae)	Fungus	Diuretic, sedative; oliguria, insomnia, tachycardia, gastrointestinal disorders

Appendix

Continued

COMMON NAME	SCIENTIFIC NAME (Family Name)	PART USED	MEDICAL PROPERTIES
Inula	*Inula japonica* Thunb.; *I. britannica* L. (Compositae)	Flower	Expectorant, stomachic
Jujube	*Zizyphus sativa* Gaertn. (Rhamnaceae)	Fruit	Nutritive tonic, sedative in insomnia; neurasthenia,
Licorice	*Glycyrrhiza uralensis* Fisch. (Leguminosae)	Root	Dumulcent, expectorant, pharyngeal irritation, cough, emollient in peptic ulcer
Longan	*Euphoria longan* (Lour.) Steud. (Sapindaceae)	Aril	Nutritive tonic in neurasthenia, insomnia
Lycium fruit	*Lycium chinense* Mill. (Solanaceae)	Fruit	Nutritive tonic in diabetes mellitus, pulmonary tuberculosis
Magnolia bark	*Magnolia officinalis* Rehd. et Wils. (Magnoliaceae)	Bark	Antispasmodic, stomachic in spastic gastritis, peptic ulcer, diarrhea, vomiting; antiseptic in typhoid fever, malaria
Ma-huang	*Ephedra sinica* Stapf (Ephedraceae)	Stem	Bronchial asthma, hay fever, trachitis
Mentha	*Mentha arvensis* L. var. *piperascens* Malinv. (Labiatae)	Leaves	Stomachic, carminative, stimulant, diaphoretic
Mirabilitum	Mirabilitum	Mineral	Cathartic, diuretic
Morinda	*Morinda officinalis* How (Rubiaceae)	Root	Impotence; antirheumatic
Moutan	*Paeonia moutan* Sims. (Ranunculaceae)	Root bark	Antipyretic, emmenagogue; infections of the digestive tract
Ostrea	*Ostrea gigas* Thunb.;	Shell	Hyperchlorhydria

Continued

COMMON NAME	SCIENTIFIC NAME (Family Name)	PART USED	MEDICAL PROPERTIES
	O. talienwhanensis Crosse; *O. rivularis* Gould (Ostreidae)		
Paeonia	*Paeonia lactiflora* Pall. *P. albiflora* Pall. (Ranunculaceae)	Root	Gastric disorders; intestinal antiseptic, expectorant, emmenagogue
Perilla	*Perilla frutescens* Britt. (Labiatae)	Leaves	Antitussive, stomachic, antiseptic
Persica	*Prunus persica* (L.) Batsch (Rosaceae)	Seed	Antitussive, sedative in hypertension
Phellodendron	*Phellodendron amurense* Rupr. (Rutaceae)	Bark	Stomachic; antiseptic in typhoid fever, dysentery, enteritis, diarrhia stomatitis, hepatitis, cystitis, urethritis; antiphlogistic in skin diseases; conjunctivitis
Pinellia	*Pinellia ternata* (Thunb.) Breit. (Araceae)	Tuber	Antiemetic, sedative, antitussive in nausea, pharyngalgia, singultus; chronic gastritis
Platycodon	*Platycodon grandiflorum* A. DC. (Campanulaceae)	Root	Expectorant
Polygala	*Polygala tenuifolia* Willd. (Polygalaceae)	Root	Expectorant, cardiotionic, renal tonic
Polyporus	*Grifola umbellata* Pilat. (Polyporaceae)	Fungus	Arrests local hemmorrhages
Rehmannia	*Rehmannia glutinosa* Libosch. (Scrophulariaceae)	Rhizome	Cardiotonic, diuretic, hemostatic in diabetes mellitus
Rhubarb	*Rheum palmatum* L.	Rhizome	Stomachic in gastritis,

Appendix

Continued

COMMON NAME	SCIENTIFIC NAME (Family Name)	PART USED	MEDICAL PROPERTIES
	R. officinale Baill. (Polygonaceae)		catarrh, and diarrhea
Schizandra	*Schizandra chinensis* Baill. (Magnoliaceae)	Fruit	Tonic, stimulant, antitussive
Schizonepeta	*Schizonepeta tenuifolia* Briq. (Labiatae)	Whole herb	Diaphoretic, antipyretic
Scute	*Scutellaria baicalensis* Georgi (Labiatae)	Root	Stomachic, antiphyretic, expectorant; used for dysentery, diarrhea, hypertension, mastitis, jaundice
Sesame	*Sesamum indicum* L. (Pedaliaceae) *Linum usitatissimum* L. (Linaceae)	Seed	Lenitive in scybalous constipation; nutritive tonic in degenerative neuritis, neuroparalysis
Siler	*Siler divaricatum* Benth. et Hook *Ledebouriella seseloides* Wolff. (Umbelliferae)	Root	Antipyretic, analgesic
Sophora	*Sophora flavescens* Ait. (Leguminosae)	Root	Bitter stomachic astringent in dysentery, enterorrhagia (antiseptic purgative)
Stephania	*Stephania tetrandra* S. Moore (Menispermaceae)	Root	Antipyretic, diuretic, analgesic; arthritis, lumbago, myalgia
Talc	Native Hydrous Magnesium Silicate, $3MgO \cdot 4SiO_2 \cdot H_2O$	Mineral	Antiphlogistic, hemostatic, diuretic
Tang-kuei	*Angelica sinensis* Diels (Umbelliferae)	Root	Emmenagogue, sedative, analgesic
Tu-huo	*Angelica laxiflora* Diels (Umbelliferae)	Root	Antispasmodic, analgesic, diaphoretic, diuretic
Zizyphus	*Zizyphus jujube* Mill. *Z. sativa* var. *spinosa* (Rhamnaceae)	Seed	Nutritive tonic, sedative; insomnia, neurasthenia

Index of Herbal Remedies

Note: Some remedies treat more than one ailment; therefore, many formulas appear more than once.